The Insomnia

Antidote

A proven step-by-step guide to sleep again.

By

Michael Pukasta jr

Disclaimer Notice:

Please note the information contained within this document is for educational and entertainment purposes only. Every attempt has been made to provide accurate, up-to-date, and reliable complete information.

No warranties of any kind are expressed or implied. Readers acknowledge that the author is not engaging in the rendering of legal, financial, medical, or professional advice.

By reading this document, the reader agrees that under no circumstances are we responsible for any losses, direct or indirect, which are incurred as a result of the use of the information contained within this document, including, but not limited to, —errors, omissions, or inaccuracies.

© **Copyright - All rights reserved.**

Table of contents

INTRODUCTION

Sleep is vital for maintaining our overall health and well-being. It allows the body the time it needs to relax, refuel, and recuperate. But, for millions of individuals worldwide, getting asleep and staying asleep may be a continual battle. Being an insomniac, I know all too well the anguish of laying in bed, tossing and turning for hours on end, longing for the elusive embrace of sleep.

In creating this book, my purpose is to share my own experience and the lessons I've received in my fight to conquer insomnia. I intend to give realistic advice, methods, and resources to anyone who is battling with restless nights. Whether you're a chronic insomniac like me or having periodic attacks of sleeplessness, this book is for you.

Over the next chapters, we'll explore the causes and consequences of insomnia, different coping techniques, lifestyle modifications that may enhance sleep quality, alternative therapies, and my path to overcoming insomnia. I welcome you to join me on this path of discovery, progress, and quiet nights.

Well without writing too much. Once again Welcome to the book "THE INSOMNIA ANTIDOTE": A proven step-by-step guide to sleep again. All the material in this book will enable you to conquer the process of Insomnia.

All the nights of staying up and all the days of constantly feeling fatigued will pass away. After reading this book, you will know not only about where Insomnia originates but you will also know how to treat it. Thanks again and I hope you enjoy this book and learn enormously from it!

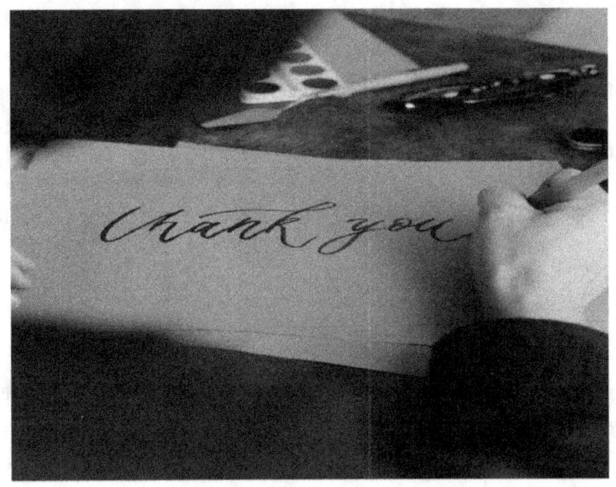

Chapter 1: The Psychology Behind Insomnia

Have you ever suffered from insomnia? In other words, do you face the challenge of falling asleep and remaining asleep at night? So what causes it?

At times, insomnia is caused by various factors, such as not getting enough rest, hunger, psychological stress, and so on. No matter what the cause is, millions of human beings suffer from the demon called sleeplessness. It robs you of obtaining adequate rest, saps your vitality, and undermines your productivity the following day.

Not to mention the adverse influence on your physical and mental well-being.

What is Insomnia?

Insomnia by definition is the problem of going asleep and staying asleep. It refers to the forms of restlessness a person suffers at various times of his or her sleep cycle. An easy sign to diagnose insomnia is when a person is not satisfied with the quantity of sleep that he or she has been obtaining.

Individuals with insomnia will experience a lack of energy, exhaustion at various periods of the day, confronting trouble focusing on duties, experiencing terrible mood fluctuations, and a low-performance level on the job. It's conceivable for insomniacs to suffer any of these symptoms after staying up throughout the night.

The human body needs rest to revitalize both the mind and body. A lack of rest in any one of them will result in weariness and various mental diseases. While they are severely fatigued to the core, they nonetheless struggle to fall asleep or remain asleep owing to different causes.

The Two Types of Insomnia

1. Acute Insomnia.

There are two primary forms of insomnia. The first kind is the kind of insomnia when you simply experience some sleepless nights.

At times, you're able to go to sleep and remain asleep quickly. Many insomniacs may not consider that they are suffering from it but the reality is, they might be experiencing Acute Insomnia.

So what is Acute Insomnia? This sort of insomnia arises from the basic amounts of stress that insomniacs are feeling at that moment. They will confront a brief time when they are not able to fall asleep due to the living conditions they're experiencing at that moment. This form of sleeplessness doesn't endure for a protracted duration.

Instead, it only occurs owing to particular variables or occurrences over a specified period.

For instance, acute insomnia could develop when insomniacs face the wrath of their employer, obtained a low mark on an exam, was rejected by their crush, or even because they're having a 'Bad Day'.

These events might lead a person to endure a night or two where he or she just cannot get any sleep. Many individuals may have experienced this form of insomnia and it tends to resolve on its own.

2. Chronic Insomnia

The second form of insomnia is called Chronic Insomnia. It's a persistent sort of insomnia that happens at least three nights per week and lasts for at least three months. Normally, this occurs when you are confronting a substantial shift in your environment, physically or emotionally. It might be relocating to a new house, losing a loved one, being in a new career, confronting obstacles in school, or having difficulty adjusting to harsher weather.

The reason why chronic insomniacs are having trouble with sleep is that they have unhealthy sleep habits without a proper sleep schedule.

It's normal in today's world; contemporary civilization has fouled up the sleep cycle with short hours of sleep. To make matters worse, most of them sleep at weird hours. They don't exercise the habit of going to bed early and waking early the following day.

As a consequence, the mind doesn't know when to shut down and would be habituated to staying up late. That's the reason why insomnia has become a prevalent issue in today's culture. What people fail to realize is that the body will not be able to function with a limited quantity of sleep one night and hope to compensate for their sleep gap by taking naps later on throughout the day.

Although this may appear plausible ́ and advantageous in the beginning, this sleep pattern is not sustainable for the long term. Ultimately, the mind and body will collapse, and you will experience utter tiredness until you receive adequate rest. The best cure is to establish a defined timetable to sleep and follow a healthy sleep pattern. Otherwise, you need to see the doctor for medication. Normally it will be related to another medical or psychiatric condition; meaning that the reason why you could be having persistent sleeplessness will be due to stress. What looks to be a routine circumstance can feel stressful if you suffer from chronic insomnia.

A restless mind and body will feel disturbed by any stimulus from the immediate surroundings.

The Causes of Insomnia

Regardless of the types of insomnia, the reasons are the same.

The difference resides in the strength of emotions a person experiences for a set length of time.

Besides that, underlying medical issues might also cause insomnia. Luckily, insomnia is curable in most circumstances.

These medical disorders might be either severe or moderate, inducing insomnia to arise at a particular period in a person's life. These symptoms include nasal allergies, sinus allergies, lower back pain, general chronic pain, gastrointestinal issues, arthritis, asthma, and other neurological disorders.

The tension in the patient's body will induce the mind to remain awake for a longer amount of time. For instance, folks who develop a cold will notice that they are remaining up for most of the night or they could find themselves waking up often. Both of these causes might result in a person experiencing a serious lack of sleep and rest. People could attempt to rest while having a cold, but insomnia will prevail.

Physical discomfort may sometimes induce insomnia since the body cannot settle into a comfortable posture to relax. Have you ever had restless nights as a result of being unable to find a comfortable position? This circumstance is usual when you encounter any pain in your body. The greatest technique to fall asleep and remain asleep quickly is to get your body in a comfortable posture in bed. It will also assist in healing and guarantee a more productive sleep. Instead, you'll find yourself in a continual fight to fall asleep and perhaps opt for unnecessary medicine if you can't get into your ideal sleeping posture.

With all of these diverse reasons in mind, we can now move on to the remedy. Yet it's just as vital to research all the components that create sleeplessness. But did you know that there are additional risk factors for insomnia? If you discover several of these hazards apply to you, then you simply have a larger probability of getting insomnia at some point in your life. Alternatively, pay attention to your health and sleep patterns to make sure that you're insomnia-free for the rest of your life.

The Risk Factors of Insomnia

The risk factors of insomnia include being a female, being pregnant or in the era of menopause, individuals over the age of forty, suffering from increased stress, suffering from depression, having night-time employment, traveling long distances when there is a time change, or have a family history of insomnia. All of these factors lead a person closer to sleeplessness. But do you understand that the majority of these risk factors are the outcomes of your choices? In most cases, people assume that they have little to no options in life, which is not true.

They may opt to take a longer vacation while they are moving through various time zones, but they didn't. They can go for a day's work, but they opted to go through the hard times of having a job at night and adjust to an altogether new lifestyle.

It is hard to cope with the risk factors of insomnia, but ultimately, it all rests on your decisions. Occasionally, you may go through tough circumstances in life. It might be love troubles, family problems, or career problems. Not only that, you can be suffering from financial or personal troubles where you are having trouble managing your career and personal life. All these will beat you up and keep you awake at night until most of the stress or despair is gone. In other circumstances, it can take longer. In other circumstances, individuals may discover answers and get through tough times relatively fast. Either way, having the correct mentality is the cure for emotions-induced sleeplessness.

As insomnia has many distinct causes and risk factors, there are many different things that you can do to protect yourself from experiencing sleepless and restless nights. Most of the time, it's simple to find out what the reasons are, but the true issue is how to overcome it and have a decent night's sleep. Life may be difficult, and sometimes it can knock a guy down to the point where he's not even sure if he can get back up.

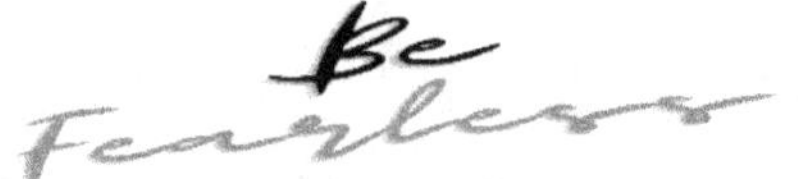

The very first step in conquering insomnia is to be brave. Do not be terrified of any events or effects that could or might not happen. Fear brings about extra stress in your life that doesn't serve you. It might simply aggravate your sleeplessness. Prevention is always better than cure. Always remember to keep calm and follow health advice to avoid experiencing insomnia.

Chapter 2: The Brain of an Insomniac

Researchers all across the globe are putting their minds together to understand how the brain of an insomniac works. They continue to look towards the characteristics of all the brainwaves and show the ideas interact over the day and night.

How The Mind Works

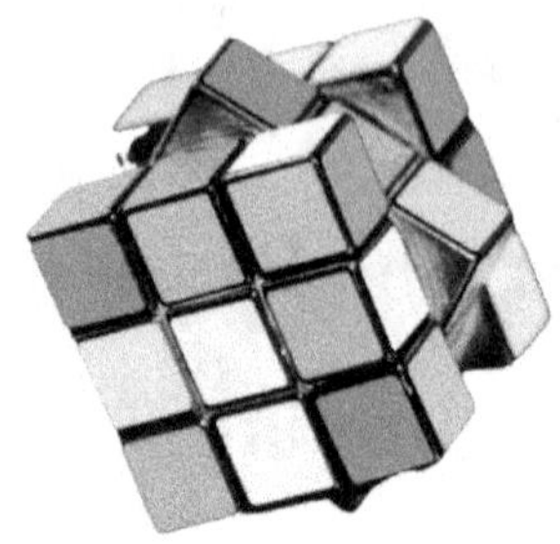

Throughout every hour of the day, the mind can adjust itself to any new scenario. Whether you're attempting to obtain food, get a drink, get out of the automobile, step through a door, or simply get some rest, the mind will continually strive to discover new methods to live and flourish. It will go through the cycle of acquiring enough resources during the day and having enough energy to recover and rest during the night.

Normally, people with a healthy level of brainwaves with satisfactory cognitive stability during the day can shut down elements of the brain's thought process during the night. When darkness falls deeper, the brain will begin to slow down and commence sleep. Your attentiveness and focus typically diminish when it's midnight. This is the reason why a person finds it tougher to finish any duties at night.

Research demonstrates that the process of the mind will naturally change throughout the day, and occasionally it may generate a severe kind of anxiety. It happens when the brainwaves become irregular and refuse to slow down owing to an excessive amount of stress over the day.

Thus, the mind will not be able to rest totally at night.

Instead, it will go through a time when the brainwaves will move exceptionally rapidly, creating more thoughts and consuming more energy in the evening. All that a person has been through throughout the day will be recollected at night. The body will then go through double the amount of energy and resources to process the ideas, and this creates exhaustion and lack of energy the next day.

The Mind And The Brainwaves

As for the mind and how the brainwaves respond to the phases of insomnia, three separate studies illustrate how the brain responds throughout the night. It has been established that the brain's learning and memory processing capabilities impact a person's sleep. The more you learn throughout the day, the more ideas and memories will be processed by the brain during the night.

Dreams emerge from one's ideas and real-life experiences. The more you encounter in life, the more you dream at night. The ability to experience a broader range of dreams enables the mind to calm down and construct hazy pictures to strengthen your memory. When you slip into a profound sleep, you tend to be in a dream state.

Occasionally, you could even experience nightmares. So it all comes down to your subconscious ideas and the type of experience you experienced.

Day Versus Night

So what's going on in the brain of insomniacs? Initially, their brain is busier throughout the night and has trouble getting too peaceful and relaxed. In one of the research on brainwaves during insomnia, scientists have demonstrated that the neurons of the insomniac's brain are more active at night.

Insomniacs tend to have a lot of ideas flowing through their head which leads to insomnia. They're experiencing a constant state of information processing throughout the whole day without the capacity to put a halt to it. Finally, they'll have insomnia and suffer the effects of not getting enough rest.

Specialists say that insomnia should not be considered immediately as a nighttime condition.

In reality, it's more of a 24-hour brain condition that causes the brain to stay active throughout the day.

Sleep has a key function in processing and storing memories. The lack of sleep will mess with your memory in the long term.

You'll have problems focusing, recalling information, and even minor details. This notion was tried out with a group of students on a brief test. One group got a full night's sleep but another group didn't get any sleep the night before. The results?

Pupils who got more sleep were able to concentrate more, and they were able to recollect their answers to the exam a few hours later. The group of students who didn't get enough sleep struggled with the exam, scored below average, and barely recollect the answers they wrote an hour after the test!

The Myths

The purpose of this experiment is to illustrate the relevance of rest to a person's attention and memory. Insomniacs aren't able to have the same degree of focus as individuals who had adequate rest. Strangely, some individuals assume that they can have the same attention span throughout the day. Just when the brain is as active at night as it is during the day, it doesn't mean that the brain can perform at the highest level.

Notwithstanding the loss of concentration, research suggests that Insomniac has more brain plasticity.

However, the research on what plasticity is and how it contributes to the states of insomnia is yet unclear. But what they do know is that the plasticity of the brain builds up throughout a person's life, and leads to different types of disease later on. Brain plasticity is the capacity of the brain to change physically and functionally in response to physical or environmental circumstances.

In most circumstances, brain plasticity permits us to absorb new information, learn new things, and continue to develop into adulthood. Yet in the case of insomnia, it destroys your brain cells and leads to brain plasticity. This leads to poor memory retention and lack of attention. not only immediately, but also over the long run. It is tougher to hold onto all the levels of focus and memory as a person becomes older.

The Brain of The Restless Mind

Another investigation was done to find out how stress and anxiety affect sleep. The purpose was to discover if a person with a stressful lifestyle suffers from insomnia, and how the brain reacts at night. And here's the result: The cognitive function of the brain doesn't alter if they experience insomnia, or not. However, insomniacs find it tougher to concentrate and process information throughout the day.

Most research demonstrates that the mind of insomniacs wanders during the night. They will have problems focusing the next day; they'll experience issues in managing their employment, academics, and even their personal life.

In other words, the mind will find it difficult to function optimally the following day and insomniacs are unable to operate at their best. Another section of the study contrasted the memory function and the efficiency to accomplish any tasks given to insomniacs and to those who had adequate rest.

Research demonstrates that insomniacs are not able to recollect most of their memories throughout the day. As a consequence, individuals experience difficulties in completing their regular responsibilities. Their heads will wander even when they're executing basic activities. For example, when it comes to cooking breakfast, folks with a good quantity of sleep will head to the kitchen, make rapid decisions, and start their day.

On the other hand, people who're suffering from insomnia will visit the kitchen, end up opening more cabinets, looking through the same items, and be unable to figure out what they should have for breakfast!

And here's the explanation: An insomniac's brainwaves are lower, and this will lead him or her to move at a slower pace and forget basic things rapidly. Additionally, as individuals continue through the day and as more activities come their way, the prefrontal cortex will begin to have fewer resources, and the brainwaves will become unpredictable. The brain will strive to remain busy, but it won't have enough energy to comprehend everything. Hence, the brain will exhaust itself eventually if you're suffering from sleeplessness.

The Gray Matter

The third and final scientific investigation is to discover the function of the brain's gray matter. The most essential thing to know about the gray matter is that it resides in the frontal lobe and governs the processes of memory and executive function. A significant loss of gray matter will occur in insomniacs when they don't get adequate sleep at night. Whether they are suffering from insomnia or having difficulties sleeping generally, they will start to develop signs of sadness or trauma slowly. Generally, the underlying cause of sleeplessness is stress.

The ideal option to resolve this problem is to see a doctor to find out what sort of medicine would be best for you.

In a word, the mind needs to obtain enough sleep and rest to have an acceptable focus. Insomnia will just force your body into overdrive mode and therefore not be receiving adequate rest. The next crucial thing to remember is to acquire adequate nutrients and sleep every night. No matter how tough it is to achieve a balance, it is necessary to have a high level of attention every day to get the most out of your day.

Chapter 3: Sleepstarved - The Real Evil

In the previous chapter, the mind was investigated to understand how insomnia directly impacts the brain. Having this disease for any amount of time will produce a tremendous detrimental influence on the mind. Alongside memory loss, insomnia also leads to tiredness, carelessness, and lack of attentiveness the following day. The mind and body both require slumber to perform effectively the following day. If there is no rest, then the gray matter, memory, and elaborate duties of the mind will break down, and insomniacs will have a difficult time getting through the day. Their mind will wander, and they will struggle to remain concentrated throughout the day.

The 5 Things You Do Every Morning

Here's a small exercise: Initially, attempt to think of all the things you did the minute you get up today. Ponder on the first five things that you did. You may turn off the alarm clock, check the phone, rise, switch on the lights, and stroll to the restroom.

No matter what your customary schedule is, you tend to complete all your regular activities perfectly. Believe it or not, you subconsciously perform all these things without giving much attention, only because it becomes a regular ritual.

Yet, when you have insomnia, you are not nearly as focused as you typically are. The mind will continue to think as swiftly as it usually would, but it does not have all the resources and energy to perform effectively. In other words, you may find it difficult to execute your first five actions in the morning and struggle to finish each activity.

One simple method to discover this is when you notice that it took longer than it should while executing these chores. The five activities that are meant to take just 2 minutes to complete can wind up taking more than 10 minutes when you didn't have enough rest.

You could even neglect to perform a job or two. You could forget to turn off the alarm, and you might forget to check your phone for any updates. Several various factors might happen, but ultimately this is merely the tip of the iceberg when you are battling with insomnia.

Damaging Your Professional Life.

During the first night confronting insomnia, you could experience a significant decline in your energy level. You could notice that it's difficult to organize the day, or you might find it tougher to remember all the information throughout the day.

In most circumstances, your daily routine may begin with waking up, getting ready for work, or even going shopping thereafter. All duties demand 100% concentration to achieve great performance and efficiency. Otherwise, you may face the music from your employer. No matter how fatigued you may feel, there are only a certain amount of days that you will be granted pity. You are only permitted to take a certain number of sick days each year. Therefore don't allow insomnia to destroy your personal and professional life. Take control and get rid of it once and for all.

In your employment, you are required to finish the duties by a certain deadline. You have to be at the top of your game practically every day, whether you are in charge of writing, researching, or packing boxes. You have to perform at your best all the time and get your well-deserved payday at the end of the month. Any rest compromised throughout the night might result in poor performance the following day.

Are You Suffering from Sleepstarved?

Everyone has a distinct sleep schedule, and experts recommend 6-8 hours of sleep every day. The precise number varies depending on the person. Some of us require more rest, others less. Yet at the end of the day, missing a few hours of sleep is always better than losing an entire night of rest. For instance, instead of receiving eight hours of sleep, you only receive six hours of sleep.

Those two hours of sleep may seem vital, but they will not do as much damage to your life as sleeplessness. Missing two hours of sleep may slow you down, but chances are, you will manage to pull it through and get all the duties done by the end of the day. On the other hand, wasting a complete night of sleep might shut your brain down. They will go spend the day grappling with basic chores.

For instance, when your employer leaves an agenda on your desk, you can read the text without difficulty. Yet recognizing what each item on the list implies is the difficult part for individuals with insomnia.

What looks to be a stroll in the park may feel like mission impossible for insomniacs.

At times, you lose focus and purpose for the day if you lack sleep. You'd be always searching for the quickest way to get through the day rather than thinking about the greatest way to get through the day. In the beginning, it could seem manageable because you're still able to get things done on time once in a while. But the reality is, it'll affect your reputation at your workplace in the long run of the low quality of your job.

Additionally, insomniacs are known to have terrible tempers and poor working connections with their coworkers.

They will notice your inefficiencies eventually. Your manager will notice that you are working at a slower pace, that you are not focusing as much, and that you do not have the necessary mindset to complete the task. That may make your supervisor dislike you, and you run the danger of losing your job. While this may seem unlikely to you right now, you should bear in mind that the possibility is quite high. Insomnia is a stressful component of life that not only may give someone difficulties in the job but also in their personal life.

Damaging Your Personal Life

As you think about your own life, think of everything important to you, things that you hold close to your heart. You might think about your wife, spouse, children, pets, or any other features. Some folks could even think about their garden or the renovation project that they have been working on. No approach to this is correct or wrong.

It's your life, and achieving success in it depends on keeping a healthy balance. Most people do their daily routine without putting much thought into it. Simple chores like making breakfast for your children, getting in the vehicle, or going out to dine are examples.

Generally, they aren't challenging jobs, but insomniacs could feel otherwise. The instant. a person's personal life begins to become off balance, it results in stressful situations, and they begin to question whether there is any way to return to a stable condition. It doesn't matter whether the tension is coming from not having the groceries in time or getting up late, a tiny bit of worry can pile into something that is out of control. Insomnia causes a large amount of stress and tiredness.

There won't be any definite ideas in their head; their mind will simply roam with random thoughts without context. The same may likewise be extended to their job life. If you are suffering from insomnia and you need to prepare your kids for school, you might miss the lunch box, fail to straighten their clothing, and the list goes on.

Always remember to put yourself first since "Self-Love is NOT Selfish". When you consistently put yourself last, you'll find yourself in a downward spiral of life, unable to realize your ultimate purpose in life.

Now is the moment to blow the lid off a big misunderstanding in our society, the idea of putting oneself first as arrogant, evil, and selfish. What they failed to realize is that if you're busy fulfilling the needs of others but not attaining your life purposes, you'd feel dissatisfied and doomed. You'd lose your drive, motivation, passion, and productivity if you journey down this route. So quit pleasing others and focus on yourself first. Only by doing so you'll have an irresistible impetus to accomplish more, and have more to give in return.

At home, you may need to maintain your home by mowing the lawn or strolling around the house to check for pests. No matter what you perform, you need to remember the procedures to execute each action precisely. The minute you are suffering from insomnia, you will not be able to recall things very well, and you will have a tougher time getting them done.

Another crucial component of your personal life is your interaction with others. Whether it's your partner, spouse, wife, boyfriend, or girlfriend, being in a relationship is work on its own. If you fail to pay complete attention to your spouse because you didn't get enough rest, then you might anticipate your relationship to grow sour. This situation will lead to fights, unhappiness, frustration, loneliness, and melancholy in a relationship. All of these emotions can go so wrong to the point where a big confrontation might need to take place.

Coping With Insomnia

It's hard to cope with sleeplessness when you have little energy left inside you. You'll feel fatigued all the time and care less about things that are occurring around you. Your mind will wander, and often those ideas don't make any sense. Life itself is already hard enough. Now, consider adding in the fact that you are not getting any rest and have to face any hurdles life presents you. How would you feel? Overwhelmed? Stressed?

You can wind up wasting time at your workplace. You might fail to cook your family meals and upset your children. You might start forgetting about all the tiny things that you usually do for your love connection. Numerous aspects of your life can go south due to sleeplessness. With all these in mind, now is the time to prevent yourself from losing sleep and achieve ideal rest every night.

Chapter 4: The Cure: Natural and artificial Remedies

Sleep is highly crucial for health. We require sleep for our bodies to recuperate and renew from our day's activities. However, many individuals either have difficulties falling asleep or just don't get enough sleep, which is where Insomnia remedies come in.

There are two fundamental categories when it comes to Insomnia Remedies.

1. Artificial Remedy

The first is the Artificial Cure. This form of treatment or medicine may be obtained in the pharmacy and clinic. They are usually recommended to attack the ailment at the cause. Artificial remedy normally costs a lot, yet it often gives speedy effects.

Most drugs nowadays are hazardous, laden with dangerous ingredients that are not safe to be eaten for a lengthy period.

2. Natural Remedy

The second form of medicine is called Natural Remedy. Humans have practiced natural medicine for millennia. This sort of remedy utilizes the body's natural healing mechanism for fighting insomnia.

It is typically less costly, but what makes them stand out is the fact that they're not as poisonous as Artificial Remedy.

Regardless of the sort of cure you pick, the aim is to help you fall asleep and remain asleep. These solutions are aimed to aid you to obtain more slumber at night. Most of these medicines will cause drowsiness, so it's better to take them shortly before bed unless it indicates otherwise. It is also crucial to make sure that you talk to a doctor before receiving any drug indicated below.

Some artificial remedies given are:

1. Eszopiclone: Commonly known as Lunesta, is a series of drugs capable of putting you to sleep effortlessly and swiftly. Studies show that Lunesta may put most individuals to sleep for an average of 7-8 hours. It's a powerful set of medications, so make sure you keep away from it unless you're able to get a full night's rest to prevent grogginess. FDA allows the medicine dose to be not more than 1mg.

Any more than that could bring upon the danger of grogginess the next day.

2. Ramelteon: This category of medications acts differently, it doesn't give unwanted effects to the users such as grogginess, drowsiness, and so on. Many medicines used to induce sleep target the CNS (Central Nervous System), lowering its functions and placing the user in a drowsy condition. Ramelteon, on the other hand, addresses particularly the sleep-wake cycle. This medicine is prescribed to patients who have trouble falling asleep. Owing to the absence of adverse effects, Ramelteon may be prescribed for lengthy usage. The medication has also demonstrated no history of misuse or dependence.

3. Zaleplon: Also known as Sonata. Most medications have a long activation period in the human body. Sonata isn't one of them.

Of all the current sleeping medicines, Sonata managed to be active in the system for the lowest length of time. In other words, this medicine leaves little to no adverse effects the following morning. For instance, if a person has problems falling asleep, a pop of Sonata pill will assist him to fall asleep without feeling off the following day.

4. Doxepin: Also known as Silenor. This series of medications are prescribed particularly to persons who have problems staying asleep. You may argue that this is an artificial treatment for the "light sleepers" who readily wake up at night owing to a minimum quantity of stimulus. It functions by blocking the histamine receptors, thus aiding your sleep maintenance after you've fallen asleep. Although this drug demands you to remain asleep for a specified period, do not consume Silenor unless you're able to sleep the complete 7-8 hours at night. The dose depends on your reaction to treatment, health, and age.

5. Benzodiazepines: Benzodiazepines are beneficial for both short-term and long-term insomnia. It has a lasting impact on the body since it remains in the system for a long period. Hence, for people who've had insomnia for a long time, this medicine may help them in their journey to complete recovery.

It's widely used to treat chronic nightmares and sleepwalking. While the impact of this medicine is persistent, you might feel fatigued and sleepy the following day. Another negative effect of this medication is that this medicine might result in drug dependence, meaning that you could have to rely on this drug to fall asleep and remain asleep in the future.

Benzodiazepines may be found in sleeping medicines Triazolam (Halcion), Alprazolam (Xanax), Temazepam (Restoril), and others.

It is crucial to have a medical examination before you use any sleeping drugs. See a doctor for a comprehensive evaluation. Please talk with your doctor about the harmful effects of any medication before picking which tablets to take. Each medicine might induce different side effects. The adverse effects might include a headache, severe allergic reaction, and persistent tiredness to only mention a few.

On the other hand, others might like to opt for natural remedies instead. You don't have to rely on drugs with harmful adverse effects particularly upon waking up. Instead, why not use natural therapies to mend your sleep pattern and put an end to insomnia?

Some examples of natural therapies are:

1. Go Camping

When the pull of the TV or tinkering with the phone keep you up late at night, it's time to take the tent and go camping. Keep away from technological gadgets and enjoy a digital detox once in a while.

Place yourself in a distraction-free zone and be conscious of your surroundings and yourself. Take this time to meditate, practice some yoga, write, recall your thoughts, or just breathe.

According to multiple studies, campers who keep away from gadgets and follow winding down rituals such as meditating or listening to music fell asleep roughly 2 hours sooner than normal. Another key factor to note is that digital gadgets lead to sleeplessness.

It is shown that artificial light sources can negatively disrupt circadian rhythms.

Try sleeping on the earth, not in your vehicle or cabin. That way, you'll become grounded and be one with nature. Regardless of what you do when camping, the ultimate objective is to relax, remove yourself from distractions and demands from people, stay away from artificial light, and be one with nature. Bath in the natural solar light and fall asleep as the sun goes down. In no time at all, you'll readjust your sleep cycles.

2. Music Therapy

Music has been utilized since ancient times to fight sleeplessness. It is a therapeutic technique that may assist to alleviate anxiety which can contribute to poor sleep quality. The biggest benefit of this technique is that it's straightforward to apply and has no negative effect.

There are many distinct sorts of music therapy and they differ in the types of neural stimulation they trigger. For instance, classical music may be a great tool for comfort and relaxation whereas rock music may bring pain. Try to opt for soft calming music that contains sounds of nature like the ocean, birds, waterfall, etc.

Numerous studies indicated that persons who listen to relaxing music before going to bed had greater sleep quality throughout the night than people who don't. So, if you're having difficulties falling asleep, this may be a remedy.

3. Power Down For Better Sleep

Sleep is not an on-and-off switch. Your body needs time to unwind and prepare itself for shuteye. Insomniacs typically find it difficult to shut off their thoughts at night. You might attempt to power down for better sleep. This strategy assists in quieting things down so that your body will realize that it's time to get some rest. To set the setting for sleep, it is vital to relax and quiet our thoughts.

For instance, if you take a warm before night, it'll induce a drop in body temperature, activating the body to start preparing for sleep. By having a warm shower, your body temperature will slow down metabolic activities including respiration, digestion, and heart rate. Your body will comprehend that it's time to slow down and relax. If you practice listening to music before heading to bed every night, your body will be conditioned that listening to music at night signifies bedtime.

It's all about habits and conditioning. Carve aside at least half an hour of wind-down time before bed to practice breathing or relaxation exercises to clear your thoughts. The purpose of this power-down hour is to notify your brain that it's time to wind down, relax and sleep.

4. Sleep In A Cool Room

Individuals who've issues falling asleep frequently have a greater core body temperature shortly previous falling asleep as compared to their healthy peers. Consequently, this group of insomniacs needs to wait for at least 2 to 4 hours before their body temperature decreases and enters sleep.

Studies reveal that the best room temperature for sleep is between 16 to 20 degrees Celsius. While you're attempting to sleep, your brain appreciates the cool surroundings.

Additionally, sleeping in a cool bedroom also assists in anti-aging. It aids in the release of anti-aging hormones known as melatonin, a potent antioxidant that battles inflammation, boosts the immune system, and prevents cognitive degradation and cancer.

There's a notion that individuals who go to bed early and wake early live longer. That makes a lot of sense given that sleeping in a cold bedroom decreases neurodegeneration and oxidative stress. I can go on and on to explain the anti-aging effects of enjoying a good night's sleep in a cool atmosphere. Yet the key to improving the production of anti-aging hormones in your body is to get adequate sleep.

And the first step to achieving so is to establish an appropriate sleeping environment by reducing the bedroom temperature. Insufficient sleep has several detrimental repercussions on your physical and mental health. Finally, it may put your life in danger. Therefore be sure to change your sleeping patterns, and you may begin doing so by establishing an optimal sleeping environment.

5. Break A Sweat (Exercise early).

It's no secret that exercise enhances health in general and sleep. However, research published in the journal Sleep demonstrates that the quantity of exercise done and when they work out make a difference. Researchers observed that women who exercise at a moderate level for at least 30 minutes each morning, 7 days a week, had fewer problems sleeping than women who exercise less or later in the day. Morning exercise tends to favorably alter our body rhythms which in turn increases our sleep quality.

Body temperature might be a contributing factor in the connection between exercise and sleep. Your body temperature increases during exercise and takes up to 6 hours to settle back down to normal. It's because colder body temperatures connect to greater sleep. Therefore it's important to allow your body time to chill down before bed.

Sleep is an essential aspect of our health and recovery. Take it seriously, and seek out the advice of a functional medicine practitioner if you can't get your sleep under control. All things take discipline and commitment. As you reset your biological clock and go back into the regular sleep schedule, you'll finally experience the advantages of restful, restorative sleep.

Chapter 5: Lifestyle Adjustment for Insomniac

In the last chapter, we spoke about the two fundamental categories of therapies to combat insomnia. Yet, these extrinsic elements could not deal with the source of sleeplessness. Yes, you may feel better after trying out such solutions, but insomnia can only be fixed entirely if the cause of the issue is removed. Otherwise, there is a great risk of insomnia relapse.

So what is the origin of insomnia? For many, the major cause of insomnia is having a bad lifestyle and sleep habits. Simple lifestyle modifications may make a world of difference to the quality of your sleep.

While not all insomnia is caused by stress, it is undeniable that people who experience ongoing stress are more susceptible to insomnia. In the case of stress-related insomnia, addressing or removing the stress will alleviate sleeplessness. As indicated in the previous chapter of this book, stress affects the quality of one's sleep which might alter his or her sleep rhythm. Hence, one will find it difficult to go to sleep at night and stay awake throughout the day.

It is crucial to manage all elements of your life in the best manner possible to ensure that you are at a healthy equilibrium. You need to make sure that you are receiving adequate sleep regularly.

Sleep has a crucial impact on your physical well-being. Insufficient sleep for a short period may make you more cranky and irritated. Long-term consequences may be serious: cardiac issues, depression, stroke, and heart attack, to mention a few.

According to sleep specialists, multiple studies demonstrated that when people get adequate sleep, they will not only feel better, but will also boost their chances of living longer, healthier, and more accomplished lives.

To combat insomnia, you should keep away from any nicotine, caffeine, and alcohol. All of these will lead the mind to become restless over time naturally. Possessing a continuous dose of caffeine will drive the mind to be more active than it is.

Most individuals require the energy to start their day, thus they choose stimulants. Caffeine is one of the most common options of stimulants nowadays to guarantee alertness and wakefulness in the morning and throughout the rest of the day. Unfortunately, they're unaware of the fact that caffeine is one of the primary causes of sleeplessness.

It breaks up the normal balance of alertness and sleep. Consequently, insomniacs should keep away from these beverages to have a great sleep. Skip that coffee break, and opt for a glass of plain water instead of coffee, which may be the reason why you are having difficulties falling and staying asleep at night.

Alongside that, putting up a sleep plan for yourself is one of the best self-help approaches for insomnia. That is a crucial step in overcoming insomnia for good. It is extremely crucial to go to bed at the same time at night and get up at the same time every morning because the body requires consistency. The body enjoys a routine. It thrives on habit. With consistent sleep and wake-up time, your body is more likely to remain on track. If you can, avoid alternating schedules, late-night parties, night shifts, or other activities that may disrupt your sleep routine.

When you have a tough time going to sleep, try to consume a glass of warm milk. Chamomile is a traditional cure for insomnia and there's evidence that it might assist you to obtain higher-quality sleep. Not only does milk help prevent hunger from interrupting your sleep, but it also includes an amino acid called tryptophan, which is processed in the brain into a "relaxing" neurotransmitter known as serotonin. Calcium is particularly pro-metabolic, lowering stress and decreasing levels of parathyroid hormone, which has been known to have a role in sleeplessness.

Not only that, you can always adapt your daily routine to include time for yoga or meditation. There is an abundance of evidence that yoga and meditation may improve sleep patterns, and soften them substantially. Taking some relaxing time for oneself is important. These approaches may be done at home for both comfort and privacy. Your body will be more flexible overall, your mind will be more at peace, and your body will be less stressed. Strive to spend at least 30 minutes a day in either meditation or yoga. Typically meditation and yoga are best done in the early morning, in a quiet environment, and with exposure to sunshine.

For meditation, all you have to do is sit down and empty your mind. Try to listen to peaceful music to help calm you down. The moment you start to become acclimated to the thought of meditating throughout the day, the mind will be able to relax quicker at night and consequently, you will have an easier time falling asleep.

As for yoga, you can either attend yoga sessions with a group of friends or practice at home for more solitude. It will enhance your sleep in various ways. The practice of particular yoga poses will increase blood circulation to the sleep center in the brain, which has the effect of regulating the sleep cycle.

Remember, sleep is not a lifestyle choice or a luxury; it is natural and required. To find out the underlying reasons, modify your diet, have a glass of warm milk, set up a sleeping regimen, do some yoga, and meditate. Follow the bits of advice mentioned above, and soon, you'll get your great sleep.

Chapter 6: Switching Off

Fighting Insomnia

Overcoming insomnia is an uphill struggle. While you are attempting to cure insomnia, you are trying to stop your mind from being too busy at night. There is no need to be terrified of staying up for endless nights in a row and wondering whether it is all going to send. Worrying can only bring about sleepless nights. So stop battling insomnia in your head! All that you need to do is 'Switch Off' your monkey brain.

At night, you want your thoughts to quiet down to the point where you can rapidly fall asleep. Getting the correct quantity of sleep helps you to be completely aware the following day, and assures a pleasant night's rest. One of the reasons why individuals struggle to fall asleep is because their monkey brains refuse to shut down. More often than not, individuals start thinking about pointless things that serve no purpose but just impede them from going to sleep.

Switching off involves practice. For many busy individuals, the only time they reflect on their life is around night! It's fine to reflect once in a while, but not at sleep. At times, this is the biggest factor that hinders you from going to sleep.

So for people who want to think about their life, try waking up earlier to have time in the morning to do so or even schedule some time in the evening to conduct some introspection.

Stimulating Night = Poor Sleep

Another reason why individuals struggle to switch off is that they have many activities at night that are highly stimulating, forcing them to remain awake instead of feeling exhausted. Some even prefer to have caffeine at night! No surprise folks are struggling to fall asleep!

Therefore keep away from coffee, from your mobile phones, laptops, and televisions when it's nighttime. Avoid activities that cause you to think and involve physical energy at night. And most importantly, prevent 'Blue-screen' from the electrical equipment.

Never Miss Another Night of Sleep

Another method to fall asleep is to arrange your sleep. Most people don't do that. Instead, people opt to fall asleep just when they're weary. So what they should do instead is to set up their routine and arrange their bedtime. With repeats, your mind will is conditioned to switch off when the clock approaches the usual hour to go to sleep.

Following a consistent sleep routine is undoubtedly the best approach to ensure higher-quality sleep. Our bodies rely on stable sleep regimens and regularity. Although there's no one-size-fits-all approach, establishing a consistent sleep routine will undoubtedly aid in defeating chronic insomnia once and for all.

How To 'Switch Off' At Night

The first thing you should do after you have eaten supper and cleaned up for the night is switch off any of your electronic gadgets.

Having your phone or computer turned on as you are getting ready for bed can excite your brain and it will eventually impede your sleep. Admit it, your electronic devices are addicting, and you won't know when to quit.

The light will conflict with your sleep pattern and force you to stay wide awake. It's advisable to avoid using your electronics at all costs at least 1 hour before night.

Reading before sleep is acceptable, but not via your electronic devices. Reading a physical book as a pastime before bed helps you in getting ready to sleep. It's preferable not to read in your bedroom. You're suggested to read in another room because you do not want your thoughts to be busy in the place that you need to fall asleep in. Again, to teach your mind to turn off the moment you go inside your bedroom. If you can entirely relax when reading a book, then it's good to do it while lying down in bed. Otherwise, it's preferable to read in another room.

The next thing you might do is listen to music and jot down any kind of reminders that you will need for the following day. The music will enable you to quiet your thoughts and erase your tension away. Try to listen to music with a mellower, slower beat.

Listening to anything loud or interesting can excite the mind, and it will be difficult for you to fall asleep. For instance, you'll find yourself in a much-relaxed mood when you listen to classical music rather than rock music.

Another idea is to plan your days before sleep.

Writing down reminders for the next day helps to clear up your thoughts.

Remaining awake in bed while continually reminding yourself that you need to recall anything will keep your mind engaged.

Think of your notebook as a "dump it and forget it" vault. Simply grab a piece of paper and write a few thoughts down. It will help you relax and fall asleep more quickly.

Another thing that you might do is take a relaxing drink such as tea immediately before bed. But, make sure that you keep away from coffee, alcohol, and beverages with a significant level of sugar.

A great cup of tea may quiet your thoughts down and helps your body to relax. This is also a fantastic method to generate time for yourself. A moment to quiet down and rest. You may do this while either reading or listening to music. If you don't find joy in sipping tea, then consider eating a little snack before bed. Do not consume anything that is excessively rich in calories and difficult to digest.

Nonetheless, a small snack is excellent since occasionally, the reason why you're having difficulties going to sleep is just due to hunger.

Another approach to promote pleasant sleep is to lower your room temperature. The easiest method to achieve this is to adjust your bedroom thermostat to be a touch colder. Our body is conditioned in a way that when it enters a colder environment, it will receive a signal that it's time to rest.

Additionally, why not take a brief shower immediately before bed? Ideally, a cold shower to rapidly chill off. Instead, you might attempt to get a bed fan, or a cooler mattress, or go for a brief stroll before bed.

Any of the items stated above may be a part of your bedtime routine. Go ahead and test them out and find what works best for you and your schedule. You won't have any problem falling asleep or staying asleep again in no time.

Conclusion

I hope this book might help and advise you in reducing or preventing sleeplessness. You're free to use any methods and strategies listed in this book to guarantee a pleasant sleep. After all, peaceful sleep is the cornerstone for your mental and physical well-being.

Whether it's an artificial or natural cure, lifestyle modifications, or setting up a regimen, all things help to avoid insomnia.

So what to do next? It's time to take action today!

Find out which of these approaches works best for you and implement them into your everyday routine. Put these down and imagine how your regular day looks like when you incorporate these strategies into your routine. Just by trying them out, you may find out the ideal technique for you to overcome insomnia

Please
Leave a
Review!